Specialist Outreach Clinics
in General Practice

National Primary Care Research and Development Centre Series

Specialist Outreach Clinics
in General Practice

National Primary Care Research and Development Centre Series

Edited by
Martin Roland
and
Jonathan Shapiro

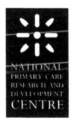

RADCLIFFE MEDICAL PRESS

© 1998 University of Manchester

Radcliffe Medical Press Ltd
18 Marcham Road, Abingdon, Oxon OX14 1AA, UK

British Library Cataloguing in Publication Data

A catalogue record for this book is available from the British Library.

ISBN 1 85775 218 X

Library of Congress Cataloging-in-Publication Data is available.

Typeset by Advance Typesetting Ltd, Oxon
Printed and bound by Biddles Ltd, Guildford and King's Lynn

THE UNIVERSITY
OF BIRMINGHAM

Health Services
Management Centre

The Health Services Management Centre (HSMC) at the University of Birmingham is one of the leading centres for health services management education, postgraduate study and training, and health services research in the UK. Established in 1972, its purpose is to promote better health by improving the quality and management of healthcare in the UK. This is pursued through research, postgraduate education, training and consultancy.

The National Primary Care Research and Development Centre is a Department of Health-funded initiative, based at the University of Manchester. The NPCRDC is a multi-disciplinary centre which aims to promote high-quality and cost-effective primary care by delivering high-quality research, disseminating research findings and promoting service development based upon sound evidence. The Centre has staff based at three collaborating sites: The National Centre at the University of Manchester, The Public Health Research and Resource Centre at the University of Salford and the Centre for Health Economics at the University of York.

For further information about the Centre or a copy of our research prospectus please contact

Maria Cairney
Communications Officer, NPCRDC
The University of Manchester
5th Floor, Williamson Building
Oxford Road
Manchester M13 9PL

Tel: 0161 275 7633/7601

Contents

1

Introduction

Jonathan Shapiro and Kevin Perrett

As the 'primary care-led NHS' evolves, one of its biggest challenges has been the disentangling of services from the buildings in which they have traditionally been provided. Conventional boundaries of care are now being eroded. More and more services which used to be the exclusive preserve of the hospital are now taking place in general practice.

This radical shift in care is not just about buildings. It is also about the changing roles of health care professionals in this new, community-based, vision for the NHS. GPs, in particular, have experienced an incredible broadening of their professional horizons. The primary care-led NHS gives them new scope to manage chronic illnesses like diabetes or hypertension or to carry out simple surgery such as vasectomies and hernia repair in their practices. GPs can also be found in some hospital clinics, so-called 'inreach' clinics, carrying out surgical procedures such as arthroscopy or gastroscopy.

All of these shifts in care involve services which are provided by primary care staff, but there is another innovation which brings hospital consultants out into the community to provide specialist 'outreach' care. It has become the subject of much anecdotal attention, with very little scientific scrutiny. But why?

The proposal for hospital consultants to work in general practice was one of the first big ideas to come out of fundholding in 1990. At first it aroused a great deal of cultural opposition as consultants balked at the idea of being more beholden to their GP colleagues. There was also a general perception that setting up new systems specifically for fundholders would create inequity and this was seen as unacceptable. It was also assumed that outreach services would be expensive, particularly when the high cost of providing consultants was weighed against the relatively low number of patients who were likely to be seen.

Against this background of uncertainty the Health Services Management Centre at the University of Birmingham convened its 1996 conference looking at the provision of outreach services. Were these developments really in the best interests of patients and of the health service as a whole?

The conference highlighted the diversity of opinions on outreach clinics. Such radical shifts in the delivery of health care often serve to emphasize the differences between professional groups and their approaches to change. Even within the research community there was no consensus as to the value of outreach clinics and the continuing debate over this issue is the inspiration behind this publication. This book is intended to highlight the key issues surrounding the provision of outreach services and to open up the debate for the future.

What does the future really look like for 'outreach' treatment? It is clear that artificial boundaries of care are preventing a real revolution in the notion of health care provision. As long as consultants are seen to be linked entirely with hospitals, and GPs with 'primary' care, and as long as the professional battles are fought over the bricks and mortar of each organization, then the whole notion of making the service more community-focused and patient-sensitive will fail to materialize. We need to include the patients' perspective (including *their* opportunity costs and not just those of the 'valuable' medical staff) and we need to follow through *all* the consequences of the different delivery systems and not merely the immediate effects on capital charges and staff costs.

It may be that there is no single answer to the question 'Are outreach clinics worthwhile?'. If nothing else, this book should raise awareness of the pitfalls and the possibilities of outreach treatment.

PREVIOUS STUDIES OF OUTREACH CLINICS

The introduction of general practice fundholding in April 1991 led to the emergence of many new specialist outreach clinics in general practices.[1,2,3.] However, several articles dating from the 1970s describe specialist outreach clinics, mainly in psychiatry but also in paediatrics and obstetrics.[4,5,6] Specialist outreach clinics in psychiatry were most common and were established as part of a move towards community-based mental health services.[7,8,9] The authors of these early articles concluded that specialist outreach clinics provided better access to more 'rational' clinical care, were a means of better communication between GPs and their specialist colleagues and were welcomed by patients. However, these articles were either opinion pieces or simple descriptive studies, apparently written by enthusiasts, and none make any formal comparison with hospital outpatient clinics. Consequently, their conclusions are largely speculative.

In the early literature, two models of specialist outreach care were described:[10]

1 the *shifted outpatient* model, where the specialist outreach clinic is much the same, apart from location, as a hospital clinic
2 the *liaison-attachment* model, where collaboration between consultants and GPs aims to provide more effective joint care.

The shifted outpatient model appears to best describe the specialist outreach clinics established in fundholding practices since the introduction of fundholding in April 1991. Although claims have been made of enhanced communication and co-operation between GPs and specialists in these new clinics, there has been no description of any attempt to use a formal liaison-attachment model.[11,12]

Despite a thorough search of the literature, only two major studies of these new specialist outreach clinics in fundholding practices were found. One was a questionnaire survey of the 15 first wave fundholders in the South East Thames Region in 1992.[2] This study demonstrated the emergence of new specialist outreach clinics in fundholding practices in that region (nine of the 15 practices had established such clinics) and elicited the views of fundholding GPs about the new development.

The second study was conducted in 1993 by researchers in Manchester. They carried out an extensive survey, by phone and by mail, of the opinions of hospital managers, specialists and GPs in 50 districts in England and Wales.[1] The authors showed a national trend in the establishment of specialist outreach clinics in fundholding practices. The findings of these two studies, and other 'opinion-based' articles, are summarized below.

Despite the absence of clear research evidence, many claims have been made about the benefits and costs of specialist outreach clinics. The most common put forward, has been that specialist outreach clinics have shortened waiting times for fundholders' patients.[1,11,13] Indeed, establishing specialist outreach clinics, in an effort to shorten outpatient waiting times for their patients, has been an important motivation for many GPs to become fundholders.[1,14] Some GP fundholders believe that improvements in services for their patients could be gained at no cost to the patients of other GPs.[15,16] However, Roland argued that fundholding 'must lead to a two-tier system if it is to work as intended, as a lever to produce change'.[17] These arguments may be becoming less relevant, both because there has been an increase in outreach clinics in non-fundholding practices, and partly because of changes in government policy which are likely to place greater emphasis on equitable provision of health care.[18]

Apart from shorter waiting times, the main advantages claimed for specialist outreach clinics have been:

- better communication and educational exchange between consultants and GPs[11,12,19]
- improved patient satisfaction[20]
- greater efficiency because of a reduction in unnecessary follow-up attendances and lower non-attendance rates.[1,12,14]

In contrast, the main disadvantages of specialist outreach clinics, apart from potential longer waiting times for the patients of non-fundholders, have been claimed to be:

- more difficult access to diagnostic facilities[21]
- reduced efficiency as patients have to attend a hospital for tests as well as attending the specialist outreach clinic[22,23]
- less efficient use of consultant time and reduced consultant cover in hospital[1]
- reduction of 'material available for teaching' in hospitals and in consultant availability for teaching.[11,14,24]

Specialist outreach clinics established since the introduction of fundholding have gone largely unevaluated. This is despite their importance as one of the most significant innovations that a major shift in government policy, GP fundholding, has produced and despite the commonly expressed concern about their impact on equity of access to outpatient services. This dearth of research evidence is also true of fundholding in general.[25] This lack of evaluation supports the contention of Iliffe and Freudenstein that 'fundholding has developed as an ideological construct, not a scientific hypothesis'.[26] It is policy-making, and not research, that is the context in which specialist outreach clinics have been established in fundholding practices. Harris rightly concludes that 'there are more questions than answers until [specialist outreach clinics] have been properly evaluated'.[27]

ABOUT THIS BOOK

In this book we describe a number of separate research projects looking at the impact and cost-effectiveness of outreach services. Each has been carried out in a different way looking at different ranges of outpatient services.

Research in this area is difficult and none of the researchers reporting their findings here would claim to have used fully robust methods for comparing hospital clinics with outreach clinics. The conclusions they reach are therefore diverse.

In Chapter 2 Kevin Perrett describes the rapid growth of outreach clinics in Sheffield, of which one feature at least is probably common to most parts of the country. In Chapter 3 Kieran Walshe and Jonathan Shapiro found clear benefits from the clinics they studied. By contrast, Mary Black and her colleagues in Chapter 5 found few such benefits and remain doubtful about the cost-effectiveness of outreach clinics. A range of potential costs and benefits are described in the other chapters.

In the final chapter, we draw some general messages from these five studies and highlight areas where more work may be required.

REFERENCES

1 Bailey JJ, Black ME and Wilkin D (1994) Specialist outreach clinics in general practice. *BMJ*. **308**: 1083–6.

2 Corney R (1994) Experiences of first wave general practice fundholders in South East Thames Regional Health Authority. *British Journal of General Practice*. **44**: 34–7.

3 Anderson P (1994) Are in-house clinics for you? *Fundholding*. **Feb 21**: 21–4.

4 Spencer NJ (1994) Consultant paediatric outreach clinics: a practical step in integration. *Archives of Diseases in Childhood*. **68**: 496–500.

5   Wood J (1991) A review of antenatal care initiatives in primary care settings. *British Journal of General Practice*. **41**: 26–30.

6   Couchman MR, Gazzard J and Forester S (1986) A joint child health clinic in an inner London general practice. *Practitioner*. **230**: 667–72.

7   Strathdee G and Williams P (1984) A survey of psychiatrists in primary care: the silent growth of a new service. *Journal of the Royal College of General Practitioners*. **34**: 615–18.

8   Williams P and Clare A (1981) Changing patterns of psychiatric care. *BMJ*. **282**: 375–7.

9   Strathdee G (1988) Psychiatrists in primary care: the GP viewpoint. *Family Practice*. **5**(2): 111–15.

10 Creed R and Marks B (1989) Liaison psychiatry in general practice: a comparison of the liaison-attachment and shifted outpatient clinic models. *Journal of the Royal College of General Practitioners*. **39**: 514–17.

11 Tod ED (1993) Should consultants do sessions in GP fundholders' practices? A GP's view. *British Journal of Hospital Medicine*. **50**: 636–7.

12 Dunbar J, Vincent DS, Meikle JN, Dunbar AP and Jones PA (1994) Outreach clinics in general practice. *BMJ*. **308**: 1714.

13 Bunce C (1992) Our in-house pain clinic is improving patients' lives. *Fundholding*. **Sept** 7:12–13.

14 Glennerster H, Matsaganis M, Owens S and Hancock S (1994) *Implementing GP fundholding: wild card or winning hand?* Open University Press, Buckingham.

15 Varnam M and Barker M (1995) GPs accept patients' vote on fundholding. *BMJ*. **310**: 1412.

16 McAvoy B (1993) Heartsink hotel revisited. *BMJ*. **306**: 694–5.

17 Roland M (1991) Fundholding and cash limits in primary care: blight or blessing? *BMJ*. **303**: 171–2.

18 Audit Commission (1996) *What the doctor ordered: a study of GP fundholders in England and Wales*. HMSO, London.

19   Swash M (1993) Should consultants do sessions in GP fundholders' practices? A medical director's view. *British Journal of Hospital Medicine.* **50**: 634–6

20   Bailey JJ, Black ME and Wilkin D (1994) *Specialist outreach clinics in general practice.* Centre for Primary Care Research Report. Department of General Practice, University of Manchester.

21   Hughes R (1994) Outreach clinics: the case against. *Rheumatology in Practice.* **1**: 3–5.

22   Bailey JJ, Black ME and Wilkin D (1994) The special branch. *Health Service Journal.* **July 28**: 30–1.

23   Russell Jones R (1993) Community dermatology. *BMJ.* **306**: 586.

24   Anderson P (1994) Are in-house clinics for you? *Fundholding.* **Feb 21**: 21–4.

25   Petchey R (1995) General practitioner fundholding: weighing the evidence. *Lancet.* **346**: 1139–42.

26   Iliffe S and Freudenstein U (1994) Fundholding: from solution to problem. *BMJ.* **308**: 3–4.

27   Harris A (1994) Specialist outreach clinics: more questions than answers until they have been properly evaluated. *BMJ.* **308**: 1053.

2

Sheffield

Kevin Perrett

BACKGROUND

The introduction of general practice fundholding in April 1991 led to the emergence nationally of many new specialist outreach clinics in fundholding practices.[1,2,3] By 1994, although specialist outreach clinics in fundholding practices were believed to be an important development in local services in Sheffield, nothing definite was known about their impact. It was not even known with certainty whether any such clinics had in fact been established.

This chapter describes the extent of specialist outreach clinics in Sheffield and their activity patterns.

WHAT WAS DONE

This study was undertaken to establish the nature and extent of specialist outreach clinic activity in fundholding practices in Sheffield.

Data were obtained from a survey of fundholding practices and from the health authority's outpatient database. Data collected on waiting times as part of this study are to be published separately.

WHAT WAS FOUND

Information from fundholders

Of the 24 general practices who had become fundholders in the first four waves (out of a total of 119 practices in Sheffield) 11 (46%) had established at least one specialist outreach clinic by November 1994. There were 37 specialist outreach clinics in total, an average of over three per practice for the 11 practices involved. Most of the specialist outreach clinics were held monthly and all had been established after April 1991.

The cumulative number of reported specialist outreach clinics in fundholding practices for each of the first four years of fundholding is shown in Figure 2.1. The total for 1994/95 is possibly an underestimate as the data were collected in the third quarter of that year.

There were specialist outreach clinics in fundholding practices in nine different specialties. Figure 2.2 shows the distribution by specialty of the 37 clinics identified. Twenty three (62%) of the 37 clinics were in gynaecology, orthopaedics and general surgery.

Eight (22%) of the 37 outreach clinics were provided by consultants employed directly by the practice though none of these eight clinics were in the specialties of gynaecology, orthopaedics or general surgery. All the remaining 29 specialist outreach clinics were provided by the two main Sheffield NHS trusts.

Thirty four consultants in total were involved in the outreach clinics identified in fundholding practices. The number of clinics provided by each consultant were:

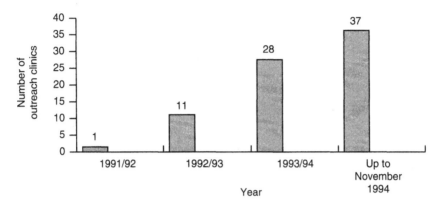

Figure 2.1: Number of specialist outreach clinics in fundholding practices in Sheffield, 1991/92 to November 1994. (Source: Information obtained directly from fundholders)

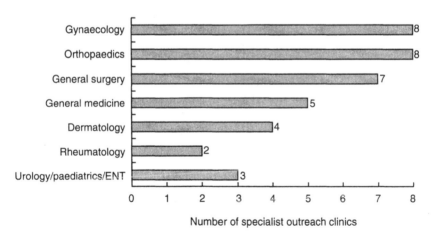

Figure 2.2: Number of specialist outreach clinics in fundholding practices in November 1994 by specialty. (Source: Information obtained directly from fundholders)

- one clinic only – 26 consultants
- two clinics – seven consultants
- three clinics – one consultant.

As some clinics were joint between two or three consultants these figures do not give a straightforward sum of 37.

Outpatient attendance data

Routine outpatient attendance data were used to compare some of the characteristics of outreach and conventional hospital clinics attendances in 1994/95 for the three leading outreach specialties – gynaecology, orthopaedics and general surgery. Fundholders had a considerably lower referral rate for first attendances in these three specialties than their non-fundholding counterparts: 73 referrals/ 1000 patients/year compared to 104.9 referrals/1000 patients/year.

There were 173 661 total outpatient attendances in 1995/96 in gynaecology, orthopaedics and general surgery. Specialist outreach clinics in fundholding practices provided 2706 (5.2%) out of 52 043 first attendances in the three selected specialties and 762 (0.6%) out of 121 604 follow up attendances.

The outreach clinics in fundholding practices accounted for 2706 (40.2%) out of 6736 first attendances for the 11 practices that had established outreach clinics (the maximum for an individual practice being 219 (60.5%) out of 553 first attendances) and 2706 (22.5%) out of the total of 12 013 first outpatient appointments for all 24 fundholding practices.

There were clear differences between outreach clinic patients and hospital outpatients. Patients who attended for a first appointment at a specialist outreach clinic in a fundholding practice, in the three selected specialties, compared to patients who attended a hospital clinic, were:

- much less likely to be classified as needing an urgent appointment (13.0% versus 32.9%)

- nearly twice as likely to be added to a waiting list for operation or inpatient admission (17.4% versus 9.4%)
- less likely to not attend or to have their appointment cancelled or changed (18.1% versus 24.8%)
- over twice as likely to be discharged from clinic (17.0% versus 7.7%)
- and, finally, less likely to be under age 16 (1.1% versus 6.3%).

It was not possible from the data available to determine whether these differences were due to factors arising from the clinics themselves, e.g. specialists may be more inclined to discharge patients when they are consulting in a general practice setting, or whether the differences were due to the casemix of patients referred.

DISCUSSION AND CONCLUSIONS

The presence of a new specialist outreach service in fundholding practices, established after the introduction of fundholding in April 1991, has been confirmed in Sheffield as elsewhere. This new service has grown to a significant size, having provided over a fifth of all fundholders' requirements for first outpatient appointments in 1994/95 in the leading outreach specialties of gynaecology, orthopaedics and general surgery. In one fundholding practice, 60% of all first outpatient attendances occurred in specialist outreach clinics in those specialties.

As the rise in the number of specialist outreach clinics in fundholding practices has been linear, it is quite possible that the number has increased since this study was conducted. Overall, however, specialist outreach activity is still small in absolute terms. Even in the three leading outreach specialties nearly 95% of all first outpatient attendances still occurred in the traditional setting – a hospital clinic.

The new specialist outreach service in fundholding practices is distinctive. Most of the specialist outreach clinics that have been established were in surgical specialties. The patients seen in these clinics in the three leading outreach specialties were mostly routine first attendees who were twice as likely to be added to an inpatient waiting list as patients who attended a hospital clinic. The fact that surgical patients who are classified as 'non-urgent' made up the majority of clinic patients supports the view that the increase in outreach clinics has been motivated by fundholders trying to reduce waiting times for elective operations (considered a high priority by GPs).[4]

As has been claimed, specialist outreach clinics in fundholding practices do appear to be more efficient in having a much lower proportion of follow-up appointments, fewer patients who did not attend or whose appointment was cancelled or changed, and a higher rate of discharge back to GP care.[1,5,6] However, it is difficult to be sure that these differences can be attributed to the outreach clinics without more detailed information on casemix. Additionally, these results support the conclusion from the literature review that specialist outreach clinics established since the introduction of fundholding are of a different type from those that existed previously.

This study confirms the importance of specialist outreach clinics as a rapidly emerging new form of care. Careful evaluation of the costs and benefits of this new service should determine their future development.

REFERENCES

1 Bailey JJ, Black ME and Wilkin D (1994) Specialist outreach clinics in general practice. *BMJ.* **308**: 1083–6.

2 Corney R (1994) Experiences of first wave general practice fundholders in South East Thames Regional Health Authority. *British Journal of General Practice.* **44**: 34–7.

3 Anderson P (1994) Are in-house clinics for you? *Fundholding.* **Feb 21**: 21–4.

4   Honigsbaum F, Richards J and Lockett T (1995) *Priority setting in action.* Radcliffe Medical Press, Oxford.

5   Tod ED (1993) Should consultants do sessions in GP fundholders' practices? A GP's view. *British Journal of Hospital Medicine.* **50**: 636–7.

6   Dunbar J, Vincent DS, Meikle JN, Dunbar AP and Jones PA (1994) Outreach clinics in general practice. *BMJ.* **308**: 1714.

3

Wolverhampton

*Kieran Walshe and
Jonathan Shapiro*

BACKGROUND

In late 1995, the Health Services Management Centre at the University of Birmingham undertook an evaluation of the outreach clinics operated by the Royal Wolverhampton Hospitals NHS Trust in the West Midlands. The Trust had run outreach clinics in some specialties for many years, but had recently expanded both the number of clinics and the number of specialties involved. Managers and clinicians at the Trust, representatives of the local health authority and general practitioners in the area wanted to compare the performance of these new, or not so new, outreach clinics with the hospital-based outreach clinics in Wolverhampton where most outpatient activity still took place.

WHAT WAS DONE

The evaluation drew on three main sources of information:

1 *routine data* collected from the Trust's information systems or other existing sources
2 *information from patients* gathered through a questionnaire survey conducted at a sample of outpatient clinics
3 *information from interviews with patients* at the same sample of outpatient clinics.

Information was collected from the Trust's Patient Management System (PMS) on the numbers of outpatient clinics, and their frequencies, specialties and locations. Data on numbers of attendances, failures to attend (DNAs), referral sources and waiting times for appointments was collated from a series of standard reports and ad-hoc queries from the PMS, all for a six month study period from October 1994 to March 1995. Information on clinic staffing levels was compiled manually by a member of the Trust's contracts staff.

Once the collection and analysis of data from existing sources had been completed, this information was used to inform the selection of a sample of outpatient clinics for further study. Four specialties were identified in which there was a significant level of outreach outpatient provision: ophthalmology, gynaecology, dermatology and ENT. In each specialty, one outreach clinic and one hospital-based clinic was chosen by the research team. The four outreach clinics selected were chosen to represent clinics in a range of settings. Once the four outreach clinics had been identified, four matching hospital-based clinics in the same specialties, as far as possible on the same days of the week but conducted by different consultants, were chosen.

A questionnaire survey of patients attending the eight clinics (four outreach and four hospital-based) was undertaken. The survey collected information from patients about how long they took to travel to their outpatient appointment, how long they spent at the hospital or clinic for the appointment, and whether they were accompanied. It also asked them whether they would prefer to have their outpatient care in the hospital or outreach setting, and how important they felt a range of factors (such as waiting times, geographic convenience, continuity of care and so on) were in their outpatient care. A total of 138 patients were approached at the clinics and asked to complete the survey, of whom all but one agreed to do so.

At each of the eight outpatient clinics visited, in addition to the patient survey, the research team sought to interview two patients. A total of 16 interviews with patients took place. All interviews were confidential and were carried out in as private a location as the clinic facilities permitted. The interviewer followed a semi-structured interview proforma and kept notes during the interview which were written up immediately afterwards.

The routine data from existing sources and the quantitative data collected through the patient survey were collated and analysed using EpiInfo and SPSS for Windows. The notes from interviews with patients and health care professionals were reviewed and recurring themes and issues were identified and noted.

WHAT WAS FOUND

Clinic activity and workload

Outreach outpatient clinic provision was concentrated in eight specialties: dermatology, ENT, general surgery, gynaecology, ophthalmology, paediatrics, trauma and orthopaedics and urology. In these specialties, outreach clinic attendances made up between 1.1% and 8.6% of all outpatient attendances. Overall, outreach clinics accounted for about 2.3% of all outpatient attendances across the Trust. In other words, although a number of new outreach

Table 3.1: Non-attendance rates analyzed by specialty and clinic type.

Specialty	% non-attendance at hospital clinics	% non-attendance at outreach clinics
Dermatology	15.0	16.9
ENT	16.6	7.7
General surgery	11.1	5.3
Gynaecology	11.4	3.3
Ophthalmology	8.0	9.8
Paediatrics	20.9	17.2
Trauma/orthopaedics	13.1	4.7
Urology	14.2	3.0

outpatient clinics had been established, outreach provision was clearly still relatively insignificant in terms of the volume of wider outpatient services at present.

Non-attendance (DNA) rates varied considerably both between specialties and between hospital-based and outreach outpatient clinics, as Table 3.1 shows. In five of the eight specialties offering outreach clinics, DNA rates at those clinics were markedly lower than rates at hospital-based clinics. In the remaining three specialties, DNA rates were similar at hospital-based and outreach clinics and sometimes slightly higher at outreach clinics. The lowest DNA rate, of 3.0% at urology outreach clinics, contrasted with the highest rate of 20.9% at paediatric hospital-based clinics. In other words, while DNA rates tended to be lower at outreach clinics than at hospital-based clinics, there were also substantial differences between specialties.

Outreach clinics had a consistently higher proportion of new referrals than hospital-based clinics, as Table 3.2 shows. Because the hospital's routine data did not contain information on the outcome of outpatient attendances, it was not possible to identify discharges and use them to calculate the number of attendances in each episode of outpatient care. Instead, we estimated the mean length of outpatient episodes of care by dividing all appointments

Table 3.2: New referral appointments as a percentage of all appointments and estimated mean length of outpatient episode (in appointments) analysed by specialty and clinic type.

Specialty	New referral appointments as % of all appointments		Estimated mean length of episode (no. of appointments)	
	Hospital	**Outreach**	**Hospital**	**Outreach**
Dermatology	32.4	63.9	3.1	1.6
ENT	29.2	81.8	3.4	1.2
General surgery	30.7	80.7	3.3	1.2
Gynaecology	34.6	56.5	2.9	1.8
Ophthalmology	23.2	48.6	4.3	2.1
Paediatrics	18.5	42.2	5.4	2.4
Trauma/orthopaedics	23.5	69.3	4.3	1.4
Urology	29.3	44.8	3.4	2.2

in the study period by the number of new referral appointments, a calculation which assumed that the clinic's waiting list was neither growing nor shrinking rapidly. It can be seen from the table that while the estimated length of episode at outreach clinics was generally between 1.2 and 2.4 appointments, the estimated length of episode at hospital-based clinics ranged from 2.9 to 5.4.

On the face of it, this suggests that episodes of outpatient care at outreach clinics were much shorter than those at hospital-based clinics. This might mean that patients at outreach clinics, because they were seen by a senior doctor, usually a consultant, were diagnosed and treated more speedily. It could also suggest that consultants at outreach clinics were more likely to refer patients back to their GPs after giving a specialist opinion. However, it might indicate that some patients seen at outreach clinics were not in need of a specialist's care. Some patients seen initially at outreach may subsequently have been passed on to a hospital-based clinic for a variety of reasons, and this might also have made outreach episodes of care seem shorter than those at hospital-based clinics.

Table 3.3: Mean waiting time (in weeks) from referral to first appointment analyzed by specialty and clinic type.

Specialty	Mean waiting time (in weeks) from referral to first appointment: Hospital clinics	Mean waiting time (in weeks) from referral to first appointment: Outreach clinics
Dermatology	11.0	11.3
ENT	9.6	7.1
General surgery	8.9	7.0
Gynaecology	8.6	7.4
Ophthalmology	8.8	8.9
Paediatrics	3.7	6.8
Trauma/orthopaedics	17.3	13.2
Urology	10.9	6.4

It has been suggested that outreach clinics, which are commonly provided for GP fundholders, offer speedier access to a consultant opinion and are a potential mechanism for fundholders' patients to jump queues for outpatient or inpatient care. However, our analysis did not support this as Table 3.3 shows. We found that the mean waiting time from referral to first appointment was actually broadly comparable at outreach and hospital-based clinics in most specialties. There was certainly no general trend for outreach clinic waiting times for first appointments to be shorter.

The costs of outpatient clinics to the NHS and to patients

We combined information from the hospital's routine data systems with data collected on the staffing of all outpatient clinics in order to estimate the costs of outpatient care. By making an estimate of the employment costs of each grade of staff (consultants, registrars, SHOs, clinical assistants, clinic nurses and other staff) it was possible to produce the estimates of the direct clinical staff costs of outpatient care shown in Table 3.4.

Table 3.4: Direct clinical staff costs of outpatient clinic sessions, appointments and episodes of care analysed by specialty and clinic type.

Specialty	Cost per clinic session (£)		Cost per clinic appointment (£)		Cost per episode of outpatient care (£)	
	Hospital	Outreach	Hospital	Outreach	Hospital	Outreach
Dermatology	208	130	13	13	40	20
ENT	227	196	5	20	17	24
General surgery	246	163	12	19	39	23
Gynaecology	191	147	12	14	34	24
Ophthalmology	306	130	20	14	85	28
Paediatrics	194	147	18	30	99	70
Trauma/ orthopaedics	223	130	7	13	31	19
Urology	198	163	13	16	46	35

These estimates must be treated with some caution, for two reasons. First, they use relatively rough and ready approximations of the number of clinic sessions and staff employment costs for those sessions. However, there is no reason to believe this data to be inaccurate, and inaccuracies which systematically affect the costings for either outreach or hospital-based care seem unlikely. Second, direct clinical staff costs account only for the largest single part of the costs of outpatient care. Other costs, such as facilities (buildings, utilities, support services), supplies (consumables, dressings etc) and services (laboratory investigations, diagnostic imaging etc) could not be assessed within a project of this scale, and so they are not reflected in the figures in Table 3.4. Some of these overheads would affect outreach and hospital-based clinics differently, and so it cannot be assumed that these costs fall equally on outreach and hospital clinics and can be discounted for the purposes of comparison.

The table presents the direct staff costs of outpatient care in three different ways, each of which has different advantages and disadvantages. For each specialty, and for hospital-based and out-reach clinics, it provides an estimate of:

- the mean direct clinical staff cost per clinic session
- the mean cost per clinic appointment
- the mean cost per episode of outpatient care.

It should be noted that the latter two costs are based on numbers of appointments, rather than attendances, and so they include appointments for which the patient failed to attend. Since such appointments incur a cost, they should be included.

It can be seen from the estimates of costs per outpatient clinic session, that hospital-based clinics were generally much more expensive to provide. However, this is simply a reflection of the higher staffing levels at hospital clinics which permit larger volumes of patients to be seen. The comparison of estimated costs per clinic appointment are more meaningful.

While there is substantial variation in a few specialties (such as ENT and trauma and orthopaedics), in most specialties the direct clinical staff costs of an appointment were of the same order, though outreach costs were generally somewhat higher. The data from Table 3.2 are used to estimate the cost of each episode of patient care. Since outreach clinics tended to have shorter episodes of care, the cost per episode of outpatient care was lower at outreach clinics in seven of the eight specialties studied.

The costs of outpatient care are not confined to the health care provider. Patients bear substantial costs in terms of time taken away from work or other pursuits in order to attend their outpatient appointment and travel expenses associated with going to and from the location where the outpatient clinic is held. Assessing the costs to patients can be a complex business, as the circumstances of individual patients will vary widely. For patients in employment, the costs of taking time off work to attend an outpatient appointment may be directly measurable but it is harder to assess for patients who are retired or unemployed. For this reason, attaching a monetary value to patients' time is not necessarily

Table 3.5: Time spent by patients and people accompanying them travelling to and from clinics and attending clinics.

	Hospital-based clinics	Outreach clinics	Significance
Mean time spent travelling to and from clinic (minutes)	51.7	23.2	U = 31.3 p < 0.001
Mean time spent at clinic (minutes)	64.0	24.3	U = 37.4 p < 0.001

Note: Mann-Whitney test used to compare time travelling for patients at outreach and hospital-based clinics; significance of comparisons reported in the table.

feasible or meaningful. Even measuring patients' travel costs can be difficult because patients can use such a wide range of modes of transport and the costs to them are often hard to disaggregate.

For this evaluation, we examined the costs to patients in terms of time spent travelling to and from the outpatient appointment and attending the outpatient appointment. We did not assess the actual travel costs, though the time spent travelling provides a rough proxy for travel expenses. We also asked about whether patients were accompanied for their appointment, by a friend, relative or carer. In so doing we were able to assess the time costs to these friends, relatives or carers.

As Table 3.5 shows, patients at outreach clinics spent much less time travelling to and from their clinic appointment, and much less time actually at the clinic than those attending hospital-based clinics. The mean total time required for the whole process of travel and attendance for the average outreach clinic patient was 47.5 minutes, while for the average hospital-based clinic patient the process took 115.7 minutes (or 1 hr 55.7 minutes). These differences are statistically significant. There was very little difference between outreach and hospital-based clinic patients in how often they were accompanied, and just over half of all patients were accompanied by someone. Taking this into account, the average

Table 3.6: Patients' preferences for outreach or hospital-based clinics.

	% who would prefer to go to a hospital clinic	% who would prefer to go to an outreach clinic
Patients attending a hospital-based clinic (n = 98)	31.6	68.4
Patients attending an outreach clinic (n = 31)	3.2	96.8
All patients (n = 129)	24.8	75.2

Note: χ^2 test used to compare preferences expressed by patients surveyed at hospital and outreach clinics; $\chi^2 = 8.72$, $p = 0.003$.

appointment at an outreach clinic took 72.7 minutes of patient/ carer time, while the average appointment at a hospital-based clinic took 177.0 minutes of patient/carer time.

Patients' views of outpatient clinics

In the survey of patients attending a sample of eight outpatient clinics, each patient was asked whether they would prefer to have their outpatient appointment at a hospital-based clinic or at an outreach clinic. From our interviews with health care professionals and patients it appeared that patients were not usually offered a choice of hospital or outreach service provision, so there was no reason why their presence at one or other type of clinic should indicate their preference.

As Table 3.6 above shows, about three quarters of all patients surveyed indicated that they would prefer to attend an outreach clinic, while a quarter would prefer a hospital-based clinic.

However, there was an interesting difference between the responses of patients surveyed at the hospital clinics visited and those surveyed at outreach clinics. Very few, if any, of the patients surveyed at hospital-based clinics had any experience of outreach clinics on which to base their expressed preference. Nevertheless, over two-thirds of them felt they would prefer to attend an outreach clinic, even though it was an unfamiliar form of service provision. In contrast, patients who were surveyed at outreach clinics had usually attended some form of hospital outpatient appointment in the past, either in their own right or accompanying someone else. They therefore had experience of outpatient provision in both settings. It is striking that virtually all of these patients expressed a preference for attending an outreach clinic.

As well as asking patients directly about their preference for outpatient clinic location, we explored their perceptions of outpatient care more indirectly by inviting them to make any comments they wished to about the outpatient clinic they had just attended. In fact, 52 of the 137 patients taking part in the survey made some form of comment.

All patients' comments were classified according to whether they were positive or negative in nature. For example, a comment such as 'I found the clinic to be very punctual and nice' was classified as positive, while a comment like 'Overcrowded and noisy' was classified as negative. Some comments could not be construed as either negative or positive and so they were omitted from this analysis. Some patients offered both a positive and a negative comment, and so they were classified as both. The results are shown in Table 3.7 overleaf. Patients at hospital-based clinics were much more likely to make negative comments (and less likely to make positive comments) than those at outreach clinics. Again, the difference was statistically significant.

Patients attending hospital-based clinics tended to make positive comments about the atmosphere at the clinic, the attitude of the staff, the perceived quality of the treatment they received and sometimes the speed with which they had been seen, e.g.

'Very pleasant atmosphere.'
'Impressed with the friendly atmosphere and very clean waiting room.'

Table 3.7: Analysis of patients' comments on outpatient services.

	Number (%) of positive comments	Number (%) of negative comments
Patients attending a hospital-based clinic	17 (42%)	23 (58%)
Patients attending an outreach clinic	14 (93%)	1 (7%)
All patients	31 (56%)	24 (44%)

Note: χ^2 test used to compare numbers of positive and negative comments from patients surveyed at hospital and outreach clinics; $\chi^2 = 9.49$, p = 0.002.

> 'The clinic gives excellent service.'
> 'I have always been happy with the treatment I have received ...'

Negative comments from patients at hospital clinics tended to focus largely on waiting times (both for an appointment and when at the clinic), facilities and the environment at the clinic and the impact of being seen by different doctors at consecutive appointments:

> 'On some days when I have come here I have had to wait two hours before being seen ...'
> 'The only thing I am not happy about is when the consultant says follow up in six weeks and when I come to make the appointment there are no clinics available until 12 weeks.'
> 'Perhaps more facilities for young children – a children's play area instead of them playing with bins, scales, fire extinguishers etc!'
> 'My first visit to this hospital – I found it very confusing finding the right building.'
> 'I would find it very helpful to see the same doctor each time (it is very unnerving to swap).'

Patients at outreach clinics almost all made positive comments. Unsurprisingly, given the nature of the survey and the setting of the clinic, these tended to focus on the advantages of the outreach clinic in comparison with their past experiences of hospital-based clinics:

'Much less intimidating than a large hospital.'
'Find it more convenient to go to GP surgery.'
'Ideal way to see a specialist. No waiting or queuing like at hospital. Thank you.'
'Quite impressed. Much quicker than hospital appointment. 10 out of 10.'
'The clinic appears to work very well. I rarely have to wait long and generally the service is professional, quick and efficient. Seeing the same specialist every visit is important.'

Only one outreach clinic patient made a negative comment, which concerned the length of time he or she had waited for the appointment at the clinic because a previous one had been cancelled.

In parallel with the questionnaire survey, we also interviewed a small sample of patients. A total of 16 patients were interviewed, two at each of the eight outpatient clinics visited. Like the questionnaire survey, in these interviews patients at both outreach and hospital-based clinics largely favoured the idea of outreach outpatient care. A number of recurring themes emerged from these interviews, including:

• the general nature of the environment or setting for care
• its impact on patients' feelings about their appointment
• continuity and seniority of care
• convenience
• waiting times
• the organization of clinics
• the importance of the quality of care, not simply its location.

Patients, both at outreach clinics and at hospital-based clinics, tended to characterize the hospital environment for outpatient care as unfriendly and unwelcoming in many ways, and to contrast this with the more friendly and welcoming setting of their GP surgery where they knew the staff. For example, two different patients commented:

'It's much more familiar, the surroundings [at GP surgery]. You get to know the receptionists and the nurses and so on.'
'The receptionists at the hospital are not friendly, they never smile. At the surgery you know them.'

Hospital clinics were viewed as unfriendly in part because patients were unfamiliar with them, but also because they were regarded as complex and difficult to find your way around. Patients described having problems in parking and finding the right building or the right department. The hospital clinic was seen as busy and bustling, lacking in privacy and prone to error:

'On one occasion they lost my file, I was there from 9.30am to 1.30pm.'

This meant that patients often said that attending hospital-based outpatient clinics was a stressful and nerve-wracking process for them:

'It's less daunting [at the GP's surgery]. When you come here [hospital] you are surrounded by all these faces, all these people in front of you in the queue, and it's stressful.'
'I'm always more nervous at hospital. I don't know why, but I am.'
'I was really nervous coming here today. I've never been to a hospital before. I know my GP's surgery and I'd feel more relaxed there.'
'When I come here [to GP surgery] I'm relaxed. When I have to go up to the hospital I'm all on edge.'

Many patients expressed a preference for seeing the same doctor each time they came to the outpatient clinic, and for those attending outreach clinics this was often cited as a reason for preferring outreach care. Some also said that they wanted to be seen by a consultant, not one of his or her team, and this was also more likely in the outreach setting. For example:

'I always make sure I see the same GP, even if I have to wait. They may not remember me, but I still prefer it. I'd like to always see the same doctor at the hospital.'
'You know who you are going to see – the main one, not the understudies.'

Interestingly, patients did not only mention continuity of medical care. Some outreach clinic patients observed that they liked to see the same clinic nurse each time, something which rarely happened at hospital clinics in their experience. Although these themes of continuity and seniority were voiced quite frequently, one patient dissented. She said that she liked to be seen by a different doctor when she came, as it gave her the reassurance of a second opinion.

Some patients mentioned the greater convenience of outreach clinics, in terms of a reduced distance to travel, though it was rarely seen as the most important benefit of outreach clinics. Those with the greatest travel problems, such as those with no car or mothers with small children, saw the proximity to home of their GP surgery as an advantage. However for some patients, especially those in work, the hospital was closer to their place of work than their GP surgery, and so clinics at their GP surgery were not necessarily more geographically convenient.

Several patients felt that they had to wait longer, both to get their appointment at the hospital-based clinic and to be seen at the hospital-based clinic on the day of their appointment. They believed (and those with experience of outreach care reported) that this was less likely at an outreach clinic, because there were fewer patients to be seen and fewer distractions (like telephone calls, messages or emergencies) for medical staff.

'You always have to wait at hospital – it's something you get used to.'
'Everything is seen to here [outreach] much more quickly.'

Some patients spoke of the facilities available at hospital, for things like tests, investigations or emergencies, and contrasted this with the more limited infrastructure of GP surgeries where outreach outpatient clinics take place. However, patients did not seem to think that this would result in outreach clinic patients having to make extra visits to hospital for investigations to be done. Several patients pointed out that, in their experience of hospital-based clinics, tests were rarely carried out on the same day as an outpatient appointment and usually required an extra visit to hospital for the tests to be done and/or for the results to be reviewed. This meant that outreach clinics, even if they did sometimes have to send patients to the hospital for tests, would not increase the number of visits that those patients had to make. A few patients pointed to the advantages of being located in the GP surgery, such as the availability of their primary care medical records if the hospital doctor needed them, and the ease with which they could make any necessary subsequent GP appointment after seeing the hospital doctor.

Most patients did not know that outreach outpatient clinics existed, until and unless they had been referred to one themselves. Almost all the patients interviewed at hospital-based clinics had not heard of the idea of outreach outpatient clinics before they were surveyed and interviewed for this evaluation. Many of the patients at outreach clinics said that until they had been referred to the clinic, they had not known that the facility existed. Patients spoke of being pleasantly surprised and pleased to find that they would not have to go to hospital, but could come to their GP surgery for their appointment.

The final theme that emerged from many patient interviews was that it was the characteristics of outpatient care that mattered to them, rather than simply the location in which it was provided. If patients' past experiences of hospital outpatient care were bad, they were likely to prefer the idea of outreach outpatient care because it held the prospect of some improvement. However, patients who had a better experience of hospital outpatient care, or conversely had bad past experiences of their GP surgery, were much less likely to do so. In other words, it was the quality of outpatient care that patients were most concerned about, and they knew that good or poor outpatient care could be provided in either setting.

DISCUSSION AND CONCLUSIONS

It must be acknowledged that there is far from an academic consensus on the value of outreach clinics. Other evaluations, drawing on larger data sets, have produced findings which fundamentally conflict with ours. Reconciling these different views is not easy and there may be good arguments for further and more detailed research.

However, some obvious conclusions can be drawn. This evaluation left us in no doubt that the patients we surveyed and interviewed preferred outreach outpatient care to hospital-based clinic care, for a wide variety of reasons. How much weight is given to the clearly expressed patient preference for outreach is a matter for debate, but in a health service which strives to meet consumers' expectations, patients' views cannot simply be ignored. Patients liked the continuity and seniority of care that outreach clinics offered, from both doctors and nurses. They preferred the friendlier, more familiar and less threatening environment of their local practice surgery. While patients certainly wanted to be reassured that they were receiving a high quality of specialist care, they saw no reason for that care to be sited at a hospital unless it genuinely needed to be.

Patients at outreach clinics also had to spend far less of their time travelling and waiting around to see a specialist, and these costs to patients should not be discounted just because they do not appear on NHS balance sheets. Extrapolating from our data, a typical district general hospital with about 200 000 hospital outpatient clinic attendances a year uses just over 67 years of patient/carer time per annum, which represents a huge social and economic cost to society.

Though the quality of the routine data available was not always high, the study team feel able to conclude that the outreach clinics performed as well as, or better than, the hospital-based clinics on most of the indicators examined. For example, DNA rates were generally lower at outreach clinics, episodes of outpatient care were generally shorter, and waiting times for first appointments were largely the same or shorter. It also appeared that the direct staff costs of outreach clinics were not very dissimilar to the costs of hospital-based clinics. Changing the basis of costing from outpatient appointments to outpatient episodes of care made a substantial difference to the relative costs of the outreach and hospital-based outpatient care, and this certainly needs to be investigated further. It may suggest that outreach clinics, staffed by doctors of sufficient seniority to make timely treatment and discharge decisions, can actually be much more cost-effective than traditional hospital-based clinics.

Of course, some of the reasons why patients prefer outreach care are more to do with the inadequacies of some hospital-based clinics than the general characteristics of hospital or outreach care. For example, problems like long waiting times, overbooked clinics, poor waiting rooms and facilities should all be capable of improvement without necessarily shifting to outreach provision. We should also be cautious about extrapolating from the performance of a very small base of clinics. Outreach outpatient clinics accounted for just 2.3% of the volume of outpatient attendances during our study period, and while the study suggests that there are good reasons to strive to expand outreach provision, it cannot inform us about the operational and strategic problems which might be encountered in such an expansion. A genuine shift towards the use of outreach clinics in mainstream outpatient care would have to be accompanied by some painful disinvestment in hospital clinics, buildings and staff, and substantial changes to the skill-mix and training of medical and nursing staff.

We believe that those who seek a definitive and generalizable truth about the value of outreach clinics are likely to be disappointed. It seems to us that the lack of consensus in the conclusions of a series of evaluations of outreach outpatient services, suggests that the performance of outreach clinics is probably highly situation-dependent, and that site-specific characteristics like geography, clinician attitudes, relationships between primary and secondary care, the quality of management and so on are fundamental determinants of whether outreach clinics are successful or not. Rather than claiming that our evaluation demonstrates definitively the value of outreach clinics, we would more modestly assert that it shows that well-managed outreach clinics can at least match the efficiency and effectiveness of hospital-based clinics – and perhaps better them.

Finally, it is salutary to acknowledge that outreach clinics have not developed because evaluations have shown them to be good, or because hospital doctors recognized their value, or because health care managers and planners decided to invest in them. They have come about because of the dramatic shift in influence and financial muscle in the NHS over the last few years, away from the traditionally powerful acute hospital and towards the primary care physician. GP fundholders have increasingly been buying outreach care and our evaluation suggests they have been right to do so.

ACKNOWLEDGEMENTS

Our thanks to Martin Yeates and Dr Matthew Perry for their contributions to the study, and to all the staff and patients at the Royal Wolverhampton Hospitals NHS Trust who took part in the evaluation.

4

Outreach clinics

in rheumatology,

ENT and gynaecology

Ann Bowling, Katia Stramer,
Edward Dickinson, Joy Windsor,
Matthew Bond and Alison Abery

BACKGROUND

Specialist clinics in primary care settings are not new but most previous evaluations have related to psychiatric care.[1] Simply shifting outpatient sessions to primary care settings does not by itself necessarily enable GPs and consultants to influence each other or facilitate joint decision making. This is because the most common model has in the past been the shifted outpatient model, in which the specialist conducts a normal outpatient clinic in general practice premises often at a time when the GP is not on the premises and contact with them is therefore infrequent.[2] A variant of this is the liaison-attachment in which the specialist attends a primary care meeting to discuss the management of several difficult patients with primary care staff, after which the specialist sees several patients, sometimes with the GP.[3] With this model the GP continues to provide treatment for the patients but benefits from joint management plans and specialist advice on patients whom he or she does not wish to refer.

Since 1990, there has been a very large growth in outreach clinics largely led by fundholding practices.[4] Given their predicted continued growth and the paucity of previous evaluation, it is important that further evaluation should be carried out.

The results presented here are based on a pilot study of the process, costs and effectiveness of specialist outreach clinics in general practice, compared with outpatient controls. The study asked, do outreach clinics:

- improve access for patients to specialist care, by reducing waiting times for appointments?
- increase patient satisfaction?
- improve communication between specialists and GPs, and have educational benefits for GPs?

Effects of the clinics on rates of referral and follow-up rates are currently being studied by this team in a larger investigation, of which this study forms a part.

WHAT WAS DONE

Data was collected from nine outreach clinics in England, in each case using local outpatients clinics in the same specialty as controls. The same specialist ran the two clinics in seven out of the nine locations. The aim of using the same specialists' outpatients clinic as the control clinics was to reduce variation between settings, e.g. in style of clinical practice.

Three clinics were included in three specialties: rheumatology, ENT and gynaecology. The outreach clinics included in the study were selected to represent a wide geographical spread of regions in England.

In each participating outreach clinic and matched outpatients clinic, all attending patients were approached in the waiting room and invited to take part. They were given a self-completion questionnaire to take home, which included Davies and Ware's (1991) Consumer Satisfaction Questionnaire, the RAND brief impact and outcome batteries, and the 12 items from the RAND version of the Short-Form-36 health status questionnaire that make up the recently developed Health Status Questionnaire-12.[5,6,7] Specialists and GPs completed clinical sheets for the patients, as well as process and attitude questionnaires about the outreach clinic. Practice managers and NHS trusts provided process and cost data.

Other data collected included socio-demographic data, a list of health related quality of life items generated by the public (areas of life most affected by longstanding illness), and a simple visual analogue scale for the specialists' and GPs' ratings of severity of the patients' condition based on the definitions used in the Duke Severity of Illness Scale.[8,9]

One hundred and forty six (83%) of the 176 outreach clinic patients attending returned their questionnaires, as did 148 (71%) of the 208 hospital clinic patients. Each of the nine specialists returned their attitude questionnaires. Forty four (73%) of the 60 GPs in the study practices with outreach clinics returned their questionnaires. The specialists returned clinical sheets for 93% of patients and the GPs did so for 58% of patients.

WHAT WAS FOUND

All the participating practices were fundholders or multi-fundholders, all had outreach clinics in other specialties and all the outreach clinics were held by consultants. Three specialists reported that their outreach clinic was conducted in normal NHS time, three said it was done in private time and the remainder said it was done in extra NHS sessions. Neighbouring practices could, in theory, refer their patients to two of the outreach clinics but in practice this was rare. Apart from two practices which paid the specialist or hospital trust a fee per patient booked (£35–£40 per patient), the remaining practices paid a set clinic fee, regardless of the number of patients booked (£230–£540 per clinic). The practice also had to bear the costs of any investigations or procedures performed in outreach that required additional facilities, e.g. routine tests requiring laboratory analysis, referral to hospital for further investigations or procedures. The average trust charges for outpatient care in the study districts (in the study specialties) was £69 for a new referral (range £48–£89, minus one trust which absorbed the outpatient cost within the inpatient fee) and £42 for a followup consultation (range £26–£64, minus one trust which absorbed the outpatient cost within the inpatient fee). These charges included basic investigations. The costings of the clinics have yet to be comprehensively analysed, thus the costs reported above must be viewed with caution as they are crude and only form a partial reflection of true costs.

In relation to outreach patients requiring further tests/investigations in hospital, five specialists said they gave them the next available appointment (thus, in effect, giving them a 'fast track'), and the remainder said that they put the patients on the waiting list and treated them as new referrals.

All but one of the GPs said the patients they referred to the outreach clinic were patients who they would otherwise have referred to the hospital outpatients' department, rather than have managed them themselves. All except one (in ENT) of the specialists said that the casemix of their outreach and outpatients clinics was similar (the one in ENT said that he saw less acute patients in outreach clinics).

Collaboration and contact between professionals

Only one of the specialists reported having (joint) criteria/ guidelines for the type of patient to be seen in outreach clinics, i.e. those with non-acute conditions. Four of the GPs said they decided jointly with the specialist who should be discharged from the outreach clinic, and the remainder said the specialist alone decided.

In six of the nine outreach clinics the specialist was accompanied by other staff, most frequently a hospital nurse. Two of the specialists reported periodically holding educational and training 'teach and treat' sessions with the GPs in the outreach clinic. Otherwise none of the specialists had planned meetings with the GPs (communications were by letter, fax and telephone).

General practitioners' attitudes to outreach clinics

Fifty three per cent (18) of the GPs felt that their skills/expertise had been broadened as a result of the outreach clinic, 35% (12) felt they had not, and 12% (4) were uncertain. Fourteen per cent of the GPs (5) were planning to develop other outreach clinics. GPs were then asked about the advantages and disadvantages of the outreach clinic. The most commonly stated advantages (by over half the GPs) were:

- reduced waiting times for patients to get appointments
- improved accessibility/convenience for patients
- fewer non-attenders than in outpatients
- improved job satisfaction for GPs
- improved communication between GPs and specialists.

Twenty three per cent (8) of the GPs said there were no disadvantages of outreach clinics. The disadvantages of outreach clinics reported by the other GPs were:

- the increase in GPs' administration costs/time
- reduced time in hospital for the specialist
- having to make repeat appointments for patients who need tests/investigations in hospital.

Specialists' attitudes to outreach clinics

All but three of the nine specialists said that they thought the outreach clinic was worthwhile. However, the specialists reported fewer advantages of outreach clinics than the GPs. The most commonly reported advantages were:

- reduced waiting times for patients to get appointments
- improved communication between GPs and specialists
- promotion of goodwill with GPs.

The most commonly reported disadvantages were:

- travelling times for the specialist
- reduced specialists' time in hospital
- reduced training time for junior doctors
- having to make repeat appointments for patients who require tests on the hospital site.

The patients: medical condition and previous clinic attendances

There were no significant differences by site (outreach or outpatient clinic) in the type of medical condition, patients' reports of impact on quality of life, self-assessed physical and mental health status, nor with the length of time patients had suffered from their condition. However, for more of the outreach patients (65%) than outpatients (34%) the sampled consultation was the first time they had attended that specialist clinic for their condition ($p < 0.0001$).

Of all the follow-up patients, a greater proportion of hospital outpatients had been attending for more than a year (40% of hospital outpatients, compared to 23% of the outreach clinic patients ($p < 0.05$)).

Time on the waiting list and waiting times in clinic

Overall, there were no significant differences in waiting times between outpatient and outreach clinics. However, for gynaecology 53% (21) of outreach patients waited less than three weeks to see the specialist, compared to 15% (5) of outpatients (χ^2: 11.52; $p < 0.001$).

There were also significant differences between sites in the length of time that patients had to wait at the clinic before seeing the specialist after the appointment time. More of the outreach (33%) than outpatients clinic patients (12%) waited for ten minutes or less (χ^2: 8.10; $p < 0.01$), while the outpatients were more likely to wait for one hour or more (22%) compared to outreach patients (5%) (χ^2: 14.54; $p < 0.001$).

Outcome of the consultation

The outreach patients were more likely than outpatients to be first attenders and there were differences in the percentages given a follow-up appointment after the sampled clinic visit: 37% of outreach patients and 50% of outpatients were given a follow-up appointment (χ^2: 5.04; $p < 0.05$).

Far more of the outreach patients' GPs had sent the specialist the results of tests/investigations when the patient was referred. Outreach patients were also less likely to have any tests requested by the specialist than outpatients: 30% had one or more tests requested by the specialist, compared to 57% of outpatients (χ^2: 16.11; $p < 0.001$). Specialists were asked if they prescribed or suggested any treatment for the patients: they reported they had done so for 76% of outreach patients and 67% of outpatients (χ^2: 4.39; $p < 0.05$).

There were no differences between sites, or specialties, in the number of types of medication prescribed, nor were there any significant differences in numbers of 'over the counter' medications purchased.

Patients' preferences and satisfaction

All patients were asked where they preferred to see the specialist: 73% of outreach patients said they preferred the GP's surgery, 1% said they would have preferred the hospital and 26% reported no preference. In comparison, 44% of the outpatients said they would have preferred to have been seen in the GP's surgery, 22% said they preferred the hospital and 34% said they had no preference (χ^2, preference for GP's surgery: 23.70; p < 0.0001).

In terms of patient satisfaction, outreach patients were more satisfied than outpatients with:

- the length of time to get an appointment with the specialist
- the convenience of the location of the clinic
- the length of time waiting at the clinic to see the specialist
- the amount of time spent with the specialist
- the convenience of the appointment day/time
- the waiting areas and facilities
- attention given to what the patient had to say.

Patients' journeys: distance, length of time and costs

Outpatients had to travel much further to the clinic: 62% of outreach clinic patients and 29% of outpatients travelled less than three miles to the clinic (χ^2: 27.64; p < 0.0001). Patients were also asked about their journey times to and from the clinic and outreach patients reported significantly shorter journey times. Outreach patients in each specialty were far more likely than outpatients to rate the journey as 'very convenient': 71% in comparison with 36% of outpatients.

These reduced journeys and journey times have implications for patients' travelling costs and associated expenses, e.g. arrangements for childcare, time off work. For example, of all those who took time off work, 50% of outreach patients and 24% of outpatients took one hour or less off work; 25% of outreach patients and 32% of outpatients took two hours off work.

DISCUSSION AND CONCLUSIONS

As Bailey and colleagues pointed out, in relation to their earlier survey of managers and doctors involved in outreach clinics, fundholding practices have used their purchasing power to secure a better service for their patients, although this leads to a risk of developing two standards of care between fundholding and non-fundholding practices.[4] In line with Bailey *et al's* findings, the study reported here found that the most common perceived advantages of outreach by doctors were ease of access for patients and shorter waiting lists. However, waiting lists were only significantly reduced for gynaecology patients, despite both GPs and consultants reporting reduced waiting lists for patients as one of the main advantages of outreach regardless of specialty.

Few of the specialists and GPs in the outreach practices held joint training and education sessions in the outreach clinic. However, over half of the GPs felt that their skills/expertise had broadened directly as a result of the outreach clinic, presumably through indirect or occasional contact with the specialists. The GPs appeared to be more involved in the care of the outreach patients, in comparison with outpatients, and were more likely to send the specialist in outreach the results of tests. There were fewer specialist follow-ups in outreach.

The casemix of patients in outreach and outpatients was similar in the specialties studied, though a greater proportion of outreach patients were attending that specialist for the first time. There was some indication that outreach patients were more likely to be treated than outpatients, particularly in rheumatology where they were more likely to be referred for therapy. The interpretation of this is uncertain, particularly as there were no differences in health status, or impact of the condition on quality of life, between sites.

It is possible that fundholders have easier access to therapeutic services through their purchasing powers, e.g. one of the practices with a rheumatology outreach clinic also had a private physiotherapist for the patients. All patients will be followed-up at six months in order to assess short-term outcomes. This issue will be addressed in future analyses, along with the comparative costs of outreach and outpatient clinic care in the specialties selected for study.

In comparison with outpatients clinics, patients' satisfaction with outreach clinics was increased while their financial and time costs were decreased. Whether these improvements are judged to be worth the increased cost to the specialists in terms of their increased travelling times and time spent away from their hospital base, with the consequent implications for hospital patient care, other work and teaching time, remains the subject of debate. The data on true costs to the practice, the specialists and trusts, and the short-term outcomes of patients have also yet to be analysed.

The other contentious issue is that of the rapid development of a two-tier service between practices with and without outreach clinics, which may, in turn, reflect fundholding versus non-fundholding practices. Currently there is not enough specialist time to provide outreach clinics in all general practices. The recent changes in specialist training and accreditation is likely to increase the number of fully accredited specialists below consultant level, making an increase in the number of specialist outreach clinics in general practice likely. A small number of districts are trying to avoid rivalry between practices by providing outreach clinics in community hospitals or large health centres for all GPs to share within a local patch. The danger then may be that these 'locality outreach clinics' become too large and divorced from personal contact with the practices, and may develop the same disadvantages of the outpatients clinics that they were designed to overcome, e.g. longer waiting lists, longer follow-up periods.

This preliminary analysis of our study suggests that outreach clinics appear to offer small but significant improvements in the quality of care provided. It remains to be seen whether such benefits could be sustained if outreach clinics spread to a larger number of practices.

REFERENCES

1 Strathdee G and Williams P (1984) A survey of psychiatrists in primary care: the silent growth of a new service. *Journal of the Royal College of General Practice.* **34**: 615–18.

2 Goldberg D and Jackson G (1992) Interface between primary care and specialist mental health care (Editorial). *British Journal of General Practice.* **42**: 267–9.

3 Creed F and Marks B (1989) Liaison psychiatry in general practice: a comparison of the liaison attachment and shifted outpatient clinic models. *Journal of the Royal College of General Practitioners.* **39**: 514–17.

4 Bailey JJ, Black ME and Wilkin D (1994) Specialist outreach clinics in general practice. *BMJ.* **308**: 1083–6.

5 Davies AR and Ware JE (1991) *GHAA's Consumer Satisfaction Survey and Manual.* Group Health Association of America, Washington DC.

6 Scott B, Brook RH, Lohr KN and Goldberg GA (1981) *Conceptualization and measurement of physiologic health for adults. Volume 10: joint disorders. R-2262/10-HHS.* The RAND Corporation, Santa Monica, California.

7 Radosevich DM and Husnik MJ (1995) An abbreviated health status questionnaire: the HSQ-12. Update. *Newsletter of the Health Outcomes Institute.* **2**: 1–4.

8 Bowling A (1995) What things are important in people's lives? A survey of the public's judgements to inform scales of health related quality of life. *Social Science and Medicine.* **41**: 1447–62.

9 Parkerson GR, Broadhead WE and Tse CK (1993) The Duke Severity of Illness Checklist (DUSOI) for measurement of severity and comorbidity. *Journal of Clinical Epidemiology.* **46**: 379–93.

This is an abbreviated version of the paper Bowling A *et al.* (1997) Evaluation of specialists' outreach clinics in general practice in England: process and acceptability to patients, specialists and general practitioners. *Journal of Epidemiology and Community Health.* **51**: 52, and is printed with permission of the Journal.

ACKNOWLEDGEMENTS

The authors are grateful to Margaret Hall and Gerald Pope for coding and data entry, Lesley Marriott for administration, Orla Murphy and Marie McClay for assistance with following up late respondents, the patients, doctors and managers who willingly participated in the study and gave their time, the members of the study's Advisory Group and to our collaborators from the Universities of Manchester and York: Mary Black, Toby Gosden, Brenda Leese, Nicola Mead and David Wilkin. The study was funded by the NHS R&D Programme and the views reported do not necessarily represent those of the funding body.

5

Outreach clinics in dermatology and orthopaedics

*Mary Black, Toby Gosden,
Brenda Leese and
Nicola Mead*

BACKGROUND

Many general practitioners set up outreach clinics following the introduction of fundholding in 1991.[1,2,3] However, there are conflicting views about their benefits.

Despite hopes that outreach clinics would lead to improved communication between consultants and GPs, a 1993 survey found that a general practitioner was present at only 5% of outreach clinics.[1] Concerns have also been expressed by specialists about the ways in which outreach clinics can increase their workload and reduce the income of their hospitals.[3] The effect on non-attendance rates is unclear and studies of ophthalmology and rheumatology outreach clinics found that costs per patient at outreach clinics were higher than at outpatient clinics because fewer patients were seen per clinic.[4-9]

The gaps in existing knowledge can be summarized in six key questions about the appropriateness of the further development of outreach clinics.

- Do outreach clinics improve communication and facilitate the transfer of specialist skills to general practitioners?
- What is the impact on hospital services of consultants' involvement in outreach clinics?
- Do outreach clinics improve patients' access to specialist care?
- What are patients' views of outreach clinics?
- Are there differences in casemix between patients seen at outreach clinics and those seen at hospital outpatient clinics?
- What are the costs to the NHS and to patients of outreach clinics compared with hospital outpatient clinics?

WHAT WAS DONE

We tried to address these questions by undertaking a study which focused on two specialties – dermatology and orthopaedics. In 1994/95, dermatology or orthopaedic outreach clinics were held in over 10% of fundholding practices.[10]

Three consultant dermatologists and three consultant orthopaedic surgeons were recruited to the study. Each conducted outreach clinics in fundholding practices and outpatient clinics in NHS hospitals in the east, west and south of England. We intended to collect data from a single outreach session in each practice and a single hospital outpatient clinic (a total of 12 clinics). However, data had to be collected over two sessions in three outreach clinics where there had not been enough patients eligible for the study at the first visit.

All patients aged 18 or over who attended study clinics were asked to complete a two part questionnaire about their treatment, any time taken off work to attend the clinic, travel arrangements and costs. Satisfaction with the clinic visit was measured by the GHAA Consumer Satisfaction Survey.[11] A second (postal) questionnaire was sent three months after their clinic visit to patients who had completed the initial questionnaire.

Data from specialists, general practitioners and managers were used to estimate costs of outreach and hospital clinics, including costs of future appointments or treatment.

WHAT WAS FOUND

Response rates to patient questionnaires

Eighty three (86%) outreach patients and 81 (75%) outpatients completed the initial questionnaires. Questionnaires were completed by all of the consultants and six general practitioners. Cost data were provided by four practices and by nine hospitals.

Communication between consultants and general practitioners

Four of the six general practitioners said that improving communication with the specialist was a reason for setting up the outreach clinic. However, only two of the GPs had any contact with the specialist when he came to the practice and none of the consultants used patients' general practice medical records. Arrangements had been made at one practice for a general practitioner to attend the clinic every month and he commented that his skills had been improved. The other general practitioners either did not have time to attend the clinics or felt that their attendance would be inappropriate.

Table 5.1: Patients' access to specialist care.

Clinic	Median waiting times for first appointments (days)	Median total travel times to and from the clinic (minutes)	Median waiting times at the clinic (minutes)
Dermatology outreach	69.0	20.0	30.0
Dermatology hospital	97.0	40.0	15.0
Mann-Whitney U test	p = 0.012	p = 0.014	p = 0.0002
Orthopaedic outreach	61.5	30.0	10.0
Orthopaedic hospital	48.5	40.0	25.0
Mann-Whitney U test	p = 0.98	p = 0.064	p = < 0.0001

Casemix

Dermatology outpatients were more likely to have chronic conditions than outreach patients. In orthopaedic clinics, outreach patients were more likely to be listed for surgery than hospital outpatients. This suggests that there may have been casemix differences between the types of patient seen in the two different settings. Direct comparisons between patients seen in the outpatient and outreach settings, in both this and other studies, therefore need to be treated with some caution.

The effect of outreach clinics on patients' access to specialist care

Waiting times for first appointments

All six general practitioners and five out of six consultants regarded reduced waiting times for first appointments as a benefit of outreach clinics. Table 5.1 shows that while dermatology hospital outpatients waited significantly longer for first appointments than dermatology outreach patients (median waiting times 97 days, compared with 69 days), the median waiting time for orthopaedic outreach patients was longer than for orthopaedic outpatients (61.5 days compared with 48.5 days), though this difference was not statistically significant.

Travel times

Median total travel times to and from outreach clinics were significantly lower for dermatology outreach patients than dermatology outpatients (20 minutes compared with 40 minutes). The difference in total travel times for orthopaedic outreach and hospital patients was not significant (*see* Table 5.1). Only five outpatients (8%) and three outreach attenders (4%) said that cost was a problem in attending the clinic.

Waiting times at the clinic

Table 5.1 shows that significantly longer waiting times at the clinic were experienced by dermatology outreach patients compared with dermatology outpatients (30 minutes and 15 minutes respectively) and, conversely, by orthopaedic outpatients compared with orthopaedic outreach patients (25 minutes and 10 minutes respectively).

Non-attendance rates

The non-attendance rate was higher at dermatology outpatient clinics than outreach clinics (20% compared with 11%) and lower at orthopaedic outpatient clinics compared with outreach clinics (3% compared with 9%), but these differences were not statistically significant.

Patients' views

Patient satisfaction with their visit

Responses to the 13 visit-specific patient satisfaction questions were recorded on a five point scale from 'poor' to 'excellent'.

Among orthopaedic outreach clinic patients, levels of satisfaction were significantly higher than for orthopaedic hospital patients in relation to:

- location of the clinic
- length of consultation
- time spent waiting at the clinic to see the specialist.

Dermatology outreach patients were not significantly more satisfied than outpatients with any aspect of their visit but the latter were more satisfied with the time spent waiting at the clinic to see the specialist.

Eighty eight out of 90 outreach patients would have been prepared to accept a hospital clinic alternative if an appointment at the outreach clinic had not been available.

The costs of outreach clinics compared with hospital outpatient clinics

The mean total cost per patient was significantly lower at dermatology outreach clinics (£43.78) than at outpatient clinics (£63.92) (average difference of £20.14 with 95% confidence interval (CI) of £1.61 to £38.68). Orthopaedic outreach total health service costs per patient were higher than those in hospital clinics but the difference was not statistically significant. Overhead costs were higher in outpatient than outreach clinics, as expected, but the difference was not significant. In both specialties, the distribution of treatment costs was highly skewed because significantly more outreach patients were put on waiting lists for surgical procedures. This is likely to be attributable to differences in the casemix of patients in the two types of clinic.

We were able to estimate the marginal cost, i.e. the cost of treating an additional patient, at the two types of clinic. This marginal cost includes staff costs, consultant travel costs and the associated opportunity cost, but excludes overhead costs (which are fixed) and treatment costs (because of such marked differences between the casemix of patients in the two types of clinic). Outreach clinics in both specialties had significantly higher marginal costs compared with outpatient clinics: average difference of £4.17 for dermatology (outreach = £7.79, outpatient = £3.62; 95% CI of difference = £3.24 to £5.09); average difference of £9.59 for orthopaedics (outreach = £15.68, outpatient = £6.09; 95% CI of difference = £4.98 to £14.19). This was due to the fact that outreach clinics were staffed solely by consultants whereas patients at hospital clinics were seen either by consultants or registrars. Furthermore, consultants were travelling considerable distances to and from outreach clinics.

DISCUSSION AND CONCLUSIONS

Outreach clinics present opportunities for general practitioner education, enhanced inter-professional communication and better co-ordination of care. However, this study suggests, as did surveys conducted in 1993, that these benefits are not being optimized because of lack of general practitioner involvement in outreach clinics.[1] A shift in the provision of services to a primary care setting does not, in itself, change the way in which consultants and general practitioners work and relate to each other.

The results of the study also indicate that outreach clinics do not *guarantee* better access to specialist care for patients and that, even where access is significantly better (as was the case for dermatology outreach patients), this may not be a benefit which patients particularly value. Patients were less concerned about the location of their consultation with the specialist than with the technical and interpersonal aspects of their consultation, echoing the findings of a meta-analysis of the literature on patients' satisfaction with medical care.[12]

Expanding the outreach clinic commitments of consultants may have serious implications. In this study, the opportunity cost of consultants' absence from their hospital base amounted only to a small proportion of consultants' working week. However, this does represent a lost opportunity in terms of time spent potentially seeing more patients in association with training of junior staff. These opportunity costs would increase with any further expansion of consultants' outreach clinic workload and could lead to a decline in the quality of outpatient care due to increased absence from their hospital base. Our results suggest that once overhead and treatment costs are excluded, the marginal cost is greater per patient in outreach clinics (as found in previous studies) due to the cost of staffing and the opportunity cost of consultant travel.[8,9] Although there may be some benefits from outreach clinics, widespread development of this model of care may not represent cost-effective use of specialist resources.

REFERENCES

1 Bailey JJ, Black ME and Wilkin D (1994) Specialist outreach clinics in general practice. *BMJ*. **308**: 1083–6.

2 Goodman I (1995) The reluctant fundholder's guide to... outreach clinics. *Financial Pulse*. **May 22**: 30–1.

3 Tod ED (1993) Should consultants do sessions in GP fundholders' practices? A GP's view. *British Journal of Hospital Medicine*. **50**: 636–7.

4 Tyrer P (1984) Psychiatric clinics in general practice: an extension of community care. *British Journal of Psychiatry*. **145**: 9–14.

5 Zegleman FE (1988) Psychiatric clinics in different settings – default rates. *Health Bulletin*. **46**: 286–91.

6 Spencer NJ (1993) Consultant paediatric outreach clinics – a practical step in integration. *Archives of Diseases of Childhood*. **68**: 496–500.

7 Goodwin D (1994) The case for outreach care in general practice. *Rheumatology in Practice*. **1**: 18–20.

8   Gillam SJ, Ball M, Prasad M *et al* (1995) Investigation of benefits and costs of an ophthalmic outreach clinic in general practice. *British Journal of General Practice.* **45**: 649–52.

9   Helliwell PS (1996) Comparison of a community clinic with a hospital out-patient clinic in rheumatology. *British Journal of Rheumatology.* **35**: 385–8

10   Audit Commission (1996) *What the doctor ordered: a study of GP fundholders in England and Wales.* HMSO, London.

11   Davies AR and Ware JE (1991) *GHAA's Consumer Satisfaction Survey and Manual.* Group Health Association Of America, Washington DC.

12   Hall JA and Dornan MC (1988) What patients like about their medical care and how often they are asked: a meta-analysis of the satisfaction literature. *Social Science and Medicine.* **27**: 935–9.

ACKNOWLEDGEMENT

This is an abbreviated version of Black M *et al.* (1996) Specialist outreach clinics in general practice: what do they offer? *British Journal of General Practice.* **46**: 558–61.

6

Ophthalmology outreach clinics in Barnet

Steve Gillam

BACKGROUND

General practitioners receive limited exposure to ophthalmology during their vocational training. There is plenty of evidence that GPs lack confidence in dealing with all but minor ophthalmological problems.[1] Many of their referrals to hospital outpatient departments are discharged following the first visit.

Outpatient throughput can be increased in various ways. However, ophthalmology is a 'shortage specialty' and increasing the numbers of consultant ophthalmologists is unlikely to be the answer. There is a need for supply side solutions to try and reduce the burden on ophthalmological outpatients departments.

In Barnet, an energetic consultant ophthalmologist undertook a feasibility study of outreach to three practices.[2] She sought to extend this with an ophthalmic medical practitioner (OMP). OMPs receive a more limited medical training in comparison to their surgically trained colleagues. They are a declining breed seeking a new role. This chapter describes an evaluation of one model of ophthalmological outreach in terms of its impact on general practitioners, their use of secondary ophthalmological services, patients' views and costs.

WHAT WAS DONE

The scheme was open to all 85 practices on the patch and 18 practices expressed interest. Although the local medical committee had expressed reservations about a controlled trial, there was some attempt to match self-selecting practices with controls using size of practice, number of partners, distance from local provider units and the socio-economic profile of patient populations. The practices received monthly visits from the outreach team that comprised an OMP and a specialist nurse. They saw 10 to 12 patients in a morning session plus follow-ups where necessary and in the afternoon, they undertook occasional minor operations. Booking and appointments were managed by practice reception staff. Both practices' nurses and doctors were offered educational opportunities to sit in with the team.

The evaluation explored the following areas:

- activity – details of the patients seen and referrals made as compared with control practices
- views of the GPs on the scheme and its educational impact
- patient satisfaction
- detailed costings.

A range of data sources including questionnaires and semi-structured interviews were used.

Table 6.1: Patient attendances/referrals from study and control practices over one year.

	Study practices (n = 18)	Control practices (n = 18)
Number of patients attending outreach scheme	1309	–
Number of patients referred to local outpatient departments	480	1187
Number of patients attending Moorfields (self-referral/emergencies)	199	330
Total patient population	125 618	125 476
Referral rates to local outpatient department per 10 000 patients per year	3.82	9.46

WHAT WAS FOUND

Activity

Only 480 (37%) of the 1309 patients seen in outreach were referred on to the local hospital outpatients department. Referral rates to hospital outpatients from control practices were three times those of referral rates from the study practices: 9.46 per 10 000 as compared with 3.82 per 10 000 registered patients.

Overall, 1988 patients from study practices were seen for a second opinion as compared with 1517 from controlled practices suggesting some supply induced demand (or lowered referral thresholds). This is difficult to assess without baseline data on practice referral rates. This was offset by the smaller number of patients who referred themselves to the Moorfields Hospital outpatient department (Table 6.1).

The age and casemix distributions in the two groups were similar with predominantly middle-aged or elderly people being seen. The most common conditions dealt with by the outreach team were cataracts and external eye diseases. Disposal patterns following the first visit were also similar in the two groups: 63% of patients were discharged, 18% placed on waiting lists and 4% received minor operations in surgery. DNA rates varied from 3% to 33% of booked outreach attenders by practice and were worse in practices serving more deprived populations.

Impact on general practitioners

Only 19 (40%) took the opportunity for learning sessions, with the outreach team spending an average of three hours with the team over the year. An increase in knowledge of ophthalmology was reported by 18 (38%) but only three (6%) reported learning new skills, e.g. how to use a magnifier, slit lamp, ophthalmoscope or testing for glaucoma.

The frequency of improvement in their ability to diagnose and manage named ophthalmic conditions is shown in Table 6.2. Unsurprisingly, a higher proportion of those general practitioners who had spent time with the team felt better able to manage one or more of these conditions compared with those who had not (42% of 19 *versus* 18% of 28).

Broadly, general practitioners' perception of the scheme was positive. It represented an addition to the range of services their practices offered and they felt the patients appreciated being seen in familiar surroundings among familiar faces.

Patients' views

The surveys of samples of patients attending outreach clinics and the local outpatients department bore out the general practitioners' positive perception of the scheme. Levels of satisfaction were high in both groups but, interestingly, of 66 patients who had attended both locations, 64 (97%) preferred coming to the surgery. They

Table 6.2: GPs reporting improvement in ability to manage and diagnose named ophthalmic conditions (n = 55).

Ophthalmic conditions	No.	% of GPs
Bacterial conjunctivitis	10	18
Allergic conjunctivitis	14	25
Meibomian cyst	12	22
Blepharitis	30	55
Corneal abrasions	7	13
Corneal foreign bodies	4	7
Stye	12	22
Floaters	15	27
Watering eyes	11	20
Age related macular degeneration	8	15
Diabetic retinopathy	8	15
Chronic glaucoma	5	9
Cataract	10	18
Post-operative management of cataract	11	20

gave as reasons the ease of access, comfortable surroundings and the familiarity of staff.

Ease of access was reflected in much reduced travelling times and distances for patients referred to the outreach team (*see* Figure 6.1). Many were able to walk and far fewer needed escorts (45% of hospital attenders *versus* 26% of surgery attenders) and 5% of outreach patients waited longer than 30 minutes for their appointment as compared with 14% of outpatients.

Costings

Table 6.3 summarizes the comparative breakdown of costs per session. Travel costs refer to additional staff travel costs and patients' costs are not included. The practice overheads incurred from monthly clinics were negligible.

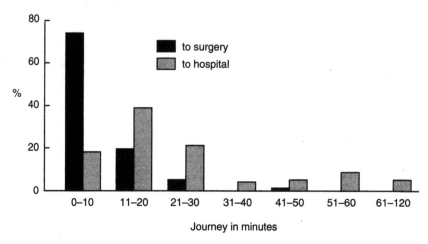

Figure 6.1: Comparison of journey times in surgery (n = 157) and hospital attenders (n = 150).

Table 6.3: Comparative breakdown of costs per session.

	Outreach	**Outpatients**
Staffing	£368.80	£282.10
Travel	£14.10	–
Medication disposables	£1.40	£6.74
Overheads	–	£11.03
Depreciation	£10.04	£97.70
Total	£394.34	£397.58
Cost per patient seen	£48.09	£15.71

Salaries make up the bulk of these costs. The total costs per session were similar. The key difference was patient throughput with approximately three times as many patients being seen in an average outpatients session. Hence, the costs of seeing a patient in the outreach clinic was three times that of the conventional outpatients department and a large increase in patient numbers would be needed to redress this. Adding the costs of those patients referred on from the outreach clinics to hospital (37%), and therefore seen twice, would further disfavour this model.

By comparison, the price of a cataract operation at the local provider unit for a fundholding practice was £1415 – the equivalent of 30 outreach appointments.

DISCUSSION AND CONCLUSION

What happened to the project? Eighteen months on, many different groups had a stake in the scheme. The general practitioners who hosted the outreach team did not want to lose the service. Local fundholders indeed wanted more. The Local Medical Committee asked that the scheme be extended to other practices and the Family Health Services Authority sought to improve relations following implementation of the new contract. The chief executive of the local acute trust wanted to increase his hospital's market share and was pushing the ophthalmologist to offer this service further afield. Her ophthalmologist colleagues, like consultants in many specialties, remained opposed to outreach as an inappropriate use of their time. The district health authority, as purchaser, was aware of benefits but concerned about the place of outreach in relation to a strategic review of acute services. Finally, the views of patients helped to justify continuation of the scheme.

Three years on, integrated health authorities have better developed strategies, and GPs have become more sophisticated co-purchasers in the primary care-led NHS. With the mix of conflicting priorities and pressures, the results of an evaluation were never likely to play the major part in the decision-making process.

Options

The early results of this work presented local purchasers with a range of options:

- abandonment of the scheme was not politically acceptable as the LMC had indicated its desire to continue
- at the other extreme, continuation of the status quo defied the evidence
- rotating participation from practice to practice might increase the learning and skills development but was unlikely to be acceptable to the current participants and was logistically complicated
- satellite clinics into which larger numbers of practices would feed referrals might be more efficient but the educational opportunities would be lost
- the service could have been left to the market but at that time there were few local fundholders.

External forces shaped the 'decision' in favour of the last two options above. With the anticipated closure of Edgware Hospital, there were plans to develop further outreach clinics. However, the bulk of the contract for ophthalmology services passed to the Royal Free Hospital where consultants were averse to outreach clinics and, therefore, no further clinics were established. The ophthalmologist who had promoted the outreach clinics moved to another hospital where she has developed her ideas on a larger scale.

What could have been done better or differently?

Provision of services like these could be made conditional upon some form of educational exchange, possibly involving the practice nurse rather than the doctor. The key question concerns cost effectiveness rather than cost efficiency. The scheme was expensive but may have addressed previously unmet needs, e.g. among elderly patients whom doctors reported would not otherwise have received a second opinion. To properly assess cost effectiveness, the ideal study would be a randomized controlled trial including before and after community-based surveys examining the prevalence and course of different ophthalmological conditions. It would take into account patient costs (as well as professionals' costs), analyze outcomes as well as activity and look in greater detail at casemix. Such a study is unlikely to report in the near future.

Conclusion

Care should be taken in extrapolating findings beyond this model in this specialty on this site but the study found that:

1   a practice-based ophthalmological outreach service could provide an effective filter, reducing referrals to hospital
2   this model was of educational benefit to only a minority of general practitioners
3   the service was popular with patients and doctors
4   the cost per patient seen in general practice was three times the cost per patient seen in a traditional outpatients setting although the overall costs per clinic were similar
5   once established, a new service may be difficult to discontinue.

REFERENCES

1   Featherstone PI, James C, Hall MS and William A (1992) General practitioners' confidence in diagnosing and managing eye conditions: a survey in South Devon. *British Journal of General Practice.* **42**: 21–4.

2   Vafidis G and Wormald R (1992) *A pilot study of consultant-based outreach.* Paper presented at annual conference. British College of Ophthalmologists, London.

3   Gillam S, Ball M, Prasad M, Dunne H, Glen S and Vafidis G (1995) Investigation of benefits and costs of an ophthalmic outreach clinic in general practice. *British Journal of General Practice.* **45**: 649–52.

ACKNOWLEDGEMENTS

I am grateful to Michael Ball, Madhu Prasad and Gillian Vafidis who collaborated on the original study.[3]

7

Conclusions and key issues for the future

Nicola Mead, Toby Gosden and Martin Roland

Shifting hospital outpatient resources into the community is part of the move towards a primary care-led NHS although outreach clinics differ from other initiatives (such as minor surgery performed in general practice) in that they represent a locational shift of secondary care services to primary care settings, rather than a change in the personnel who actually provide those services. What are the advantages of such a relocation? What are the disadvantages? Do the benefits outweigh the costs or *vice versa*? These are some of the key questions which need to be addressed.

In this book, five separate groups have described evaluations of outreach clinics. They do not arrive at uniform conclusions. Walshe and Shapiro found substantial benefits from the clinics studied, whereas Black *et al.* found the benefits to be much less clear cut. Gillam's study pointed to the tensions which outreach clinics can sometimes produce. Evaluation of a complex change such as an alteration in the location of care is difficult and none of the teams reporting their findings here were able to use ideal methods of evaluation. Several found clear differences between patients seen in hospital clinics and outreach clinics, making comparisons between the two difficult. For example, differences in the types of patient seen in the two settings were found by Perrett and Black *et al.*; Bowling and colleagues found that fewer tests were requested for outreach clinic patients and, like Walshe and Shapiro, they found that outreach patients were more likely to be discharged than patients attending hospital clinics. Nevertheless, despite difficulties in drawing valid comparisons, there are some important messages which we draw out in this final chapter.

In summarizing the results of the five studies, we have used the framework proposed by Roland and Wilkin for assessing the success of a primary care-led NHS.[1] They suggest that any shift towards a primary care-led NHS should be evaluated against five criteria:

1 equitable access to all population groups
2 acceptability to the population
3 responsiveness to the needs of the population
4 cost-effectiveness
5 accountability.

Using this framework, this chapter will discuss some of the issues in the debate about the relative costs and benefits of outreach clinics.

EQUITABLE ACCESS

The outreach model of care does not alter the fact that GPs remain 'gatekeepers' to specialist services. There have always been inequities in the system as a result of variations in GP referral behaviour and in waiting times for appointments at hospital clinics. However, these inequities would be exacerbated if outreach clinics were to confer access advantages to patients regardless of need, and if some patients were to have preferential access to such clinics.

There are two possible ways in which advantages relating to access might arise if outreach clinics were not equitably distributed across practices:

1 if waiting times for first appointments are consistently lower for outreach than for equivalent hospital clinics so that patients referred to the former are seen more quickly than they otherwise would be
2 if GPs with in-house clinics have lower referral thresholds so that more patients are seen at those clinics than would otherwise be seen at equivalent hospital clinics.

Waiting times for first appointments

Neither Walshe and Shapiro, nor Black *et al.* found consistently reduced waiting times for outreach clinics, though Bowling and colleagues found reduced waiting times in one of the three sets of clinics studied. Reduced waiting times had been regarded by doctors interviewed in these studies as an important reason for setting up the clinics and, indeed, the potential inequity introduced by easier access to outreach clinics has been used to argue against their establishment. The results of the studies cited here indicate that these fears were not borne out in the clinics studied, and the presence of outreach clinics did not confer major advantages to the patients of practices in which they were sited.

Referral rates

In Bowling's study, the GPs said that almost all patients referred to outreach clinics were those whom they would otherwise have referred to hospital. However, Walshe and Shapiro found higher proportions of new referrals at outreach clinics. Combining this with the fact that outreach patients were discharged more rapidly, they speculate on the possibility either that patients were discharged earlier because they were seen by a consultant, or that some of the referrals were inappropriate in the first place.

The data reported in these studies do not allow conclusions to be drawn about the effect of outreach clinics on patterns of referral, still less on whether any changes that might occur would be beneficial to patients or cost-effective. If outreach clinics were associated with increased learning by GPs, then there might be long-term benefits, though the studies cited here show little evidence of educational benefits for GPs from outreach clinics.

The issue of referral rates is complicated by the fact that the majority of clinics studied were in fundholding practices. Although studies have not shown any major overall effect of fundholding in general on rates of referral, the chances of being seen by a specialist at an outreach clinic might be greater for patients registered with fundholding practices than for patients of non-fundholders, so that any access advantages of outreach clinics would not be shared according to need across the population as a whole.[2] However, increasing numbers of non-fundholding practices are now negotiating the set-up of outreach clinics. A recent report by the Audit Commission showed that 50% of large non-fundholders had at least one outreach clinic sited in their premises, compared with 60% of fundholding general practices.[3] These distinctions are likely to become further blurred as new models of GP commissioning are developed. If there are perceived inequities associated with outreach clinics, then they may prove to be related to issues other than fundholding status, e.g. practice size.

ACCEPTABILITY TO PATIENTS

Proponents of outreach clinics argue that more locally accessible specialist care will result in greater patient satisfaction. However, this argument assumes that care which is locally based, i.e. near to one's place of residence, is necessarily more convenient in terms of travelling distance, time, cost and associated opportunity costs etc.

In the studies by Bowling *et al.*, Walshe and Shapiro, and Gillam, patients expressed strong preferences for being seen in their GP's surgery as this was more convenient and involved less travel. In Walshe and Shapiro's study, patients were also more likely to attend appointments at their GP's surgery. Their study includes substantial detail about the sorts of benefits that patients valued in outreach clinics which included the familiar surroundings, knowing which doctor they were going to see, having continuity of care from one clinic visit to another, and the efficient running of clinic sessions.

Black and colleagues drew rather different conclusions about the benefits to patients. They also found improved satisfaction among some groups of outreach patients but here the differences were modest and for some aspects of care, patients were more satisfied in hospital clinics than outreach clinics. They comment that other aspects of care, e.g. communication with the specialist, are more important to patients than the location of care.

We know little about what associations patients make between the setting in which care is provided and their perceptions of the *quality* of that care. The public associate general practice with first contact, generalist care that is distinguished from the relatively high-tech, resource intensive, specialist care delivered in hospitals. Hospital outpatients are more likely to evaluate their visit to an outpatient clinic as 'worthwhile' if they feel they have received treatment or tests which are not available from their GP.[4] However, these distinctions may become more blurred as an increasing amount of care previously provided in hospitals is provided in community settings.

Advantages of outreach clinics would be reduced if patients subsequently had to attend hospital for diagnostic tests or treatments which were not available on general practice premises. However, the disadvantages to a small number of patients who may have to re-attend at hospital may be countered by the increased chance, found in the studies cited here, that patients in the outreach clinics would be discharged from specialist care altogether. This may relate to outreach clinics being held by senior rather than by junior doctors.

RESPONSIVENESS TO LOCAL NEEDS

At the level of general practice populations, outreach clinics present an opportunity for providing secondary care services which are more responsive to the needs of patients. Consideration of referral patterns to different specialties and the age/sex structure of the practice population should form part of the decision-making process in setting-up an outreach clinic. However, supply side factors such as the business motives of the acute trust described in Gillam's study, will also impact on decision-making and may have little to do with considerations of the health needs of the practice population.

True responsiveness to local needs requires that patients' views are taken into account. There is a tension between meeting the needs for specialist care of a particular general practice population and being responsive to the needs of the wider community. At present, patients' views are rarely taken into account in the provision of new services, whether outreach clinics or other changes to care. In an unusual move, government has required evidence of public consultation in relation to the developing of Primary Care Act (1997) pilot sites.

COST-EFFECTIVENESS ISSUES

The cost-effectiveness of outreach clinics essentially depends on the balance of costs and effects compared with outpatient clinics. However, the effects cannot be readily measured in natural physical units such as blood pressure reduction (cost-effectiveness analysis), utility measures (cost-utility analysis) or monetary values (cost-benefit analysis). In addition, effects such as changes in the appropriateness of referrals as a result of increased contact with a consultant will be long term and difficult to attribute to the outreach clinic. Therefore, where the benefits of outreach clinics are greater than outpatient clinics but costs are higher, it is difficult to draw a conclusion about cost-effectiveness or efficiency.

There are problems in interpreting the data presented in this book on costs and cost-effectiveness of outreach clinics. For example, lower follow-up rates and higher discharge rates at outreach clinics could be interpreted as an indication that outreach clinics are a success. Reduced follow-up could be due to the fact that more experienced clinicians staff outreach clinics but it could also be due to differences in casemix between the two types of clinic. Patient casemix, i.e. the type and severity of presenting conditions, is therefore an important variable to consider when assessing the efficiency of outreach clinics. None of the studies reported here have been designed systematically to allow for casemix differences between clinics, nor do they address the question of whether certain types of patient are more appropriately seen in community rather than hospital settings.

All the studies which reported NHS costs of outreach and outpatient clinics urge caution in interpreting the results. Walshe and Shapiro found that direct staff costs per clinic appointment were increased in most of the outreach clinic studies but were reduced when related to each episode of care (since episodes of care were shorter). Black *et al.* found that total health service costs were higher in hospital clinics in one of the specialties studied but that for both specialties, the marginal cost of seeing additional patients was greater for outreach clinics. The costs are crucially dependent on the clinic organization and Gillam found that outreach clinics were three times as expensive per patient but only because three times as many patients were seen in each hospital clinic compared to the outreach clinics. A more detailed article on the complex economic issues surrounding evaluation of specialist outreach clinics is due to be published in 1997.[5]

The results of the cost analyses are, in any case, limited by the modest number of clinics studied in each of the evaluations and there is likely to be continued argument and debate over the cost-effectiveness of individual outreach clinics. Perhaps a more important point is the extent to which the outreach model could replace hospital outpatient clinics on a wider scale.

The view of specialists in these studies was that their present pattern of hospital work would not be sustainable if they were doing a large part of their clinic work in practices. Outreach clinics are currently largely run by consultants, whereas more junior staff play a major role in seeing patients in hospital clinics. The studies described here do not address questions about the impact of outreach clinics on the organization of other parts of the secondary care system, e.g. the absence of the consultant from the hospital base might have an effect on junior doctor training resulting in decreasing discharge rates in hospital outpatient clinics. Widespread development of outreach clinics would need to develop alongside new models of training for junior hospital staff.

A major expansion in outreach clinics could not take place without changes in specialist staffing structure or changes in the way that outreach clinics are run. The current 'Calman' changes are bringing about major changes in hospital staffing including an expansion of the consultant grade and more structured training for junior hospital staff. This may provide opportunities for developing new models of care and if there were a major expansion in outreach clinics, this would certainly need to be reflected in strategic planning for specialist staffing and training.

Expansion would also require capital developments in primary care, associated with either disinvestment in hospital buildings or opportunities to use space in hospitals in different ways. The reported studies certainly do not give a clear message whether this would be a cost-effective way to proceed. The effects of expanding outreach clinics is an important issue as the opportunity costs of closing down clinics, whether in hospitals or general practices, depend on the alternative use of the space and staff.

An important, but less tangible, way in which outreach clinics could prove cost-effective would be if they lead to transfer of skills or knowledge from specialists to GPs. In the study by Black et al., the GPs cited improved communication with specialists as a reason for setting clinics up but, as previously noted, contact between specialists and GPs in clinics is infrequent. Although Bowling et al. found the same, more than half the GPs reported improved communication with specialists and an improvement in their skills, and Walshe and Shapiro suggested that there might have been valuable contact between visiting hospital nurses and practice nurses. In Gillam's study, a third of GPs reported improved knowledge, though few had learned new skills in the assessment of eye problems. It is clear that outreach clinics are infrequently combined with formal learning opportunities, e.g. joint meeting or 'teach and treat' clinics. However, the value of anecdotal reports of improved communication, whether through corridor consultations or increased social interaction may be significant, though it is difficult to quantify. Informal communication between consultants and GPs could increase the appropriateness of referrals which could potentially increase or decrease the volume of referrals. None of the studies reported here are able to address this issue and none of the outreach clinics considered the possible use of outreach clinics as a method of training junior hospital staff in the sorts of problems that could most appropriately be managed in primary care. In future, the opportunities for outreach clinics to be used explicitly to increase the skills of doctors and nurses in both primary and secondary care need to be investigated.

It has been argued that outreach clinics could be advantageously used as a filter for hospital services but there are a number of reasons why this is likely to prove inefficient. First, patients would already be receiving secondary care when the filtering stage should ideally be the task of the GP. Second, patients may receive more appointments than they otherwise would do. Third, the consultant may end up seeing a greater volume of patients – those who would normally be seen and some attending a second appointment at the hospital clinic to receive tests or treatment not available in general practice.

There is clearly a balance to be struck between the advantages of providing responsive and accessible specialist care at an outreach clinic and the value lost as direct patient contact time is lost through travelling and there is less supervision of junior doctors left in the hospital. There are major difficulties in obtaining data on both long and short term effects which can be used to inform decisions about marginal costs and benefits. These studies do not enable us to draw firm conclusions about the efficiency of outreach clinics.

ACCOUNTABILITY

In an ideal world the incentives of the NHS managers, specialists and general practitioners who make the decisions to set-up outreach clinics would be aligned with those to whom they are accountable, namely the patients. However, in practice the situation is far from straightforward and the ethos of the internal market has encouraged providers, to varying degrees, to strive for income maximization. Purchasers are encouraged to seek out providers who can deliver the greatest health gain per unit of resource and trusts seek to maximize income and minimize expenditure. This feature of the internal market has meant that these bodies may fail to consider all the relevant costs and benefits in making decisions about which health care services to provide and where. The incentives of providers have not been fully aligned with those of patients and with the societal objectives of cost-effectiveness, equity, accountability, responsiveness and acceptability. It remains to be seen how these issues will be addressed in relation to outreach clinics with the government's new commissioning arrangements, which are likely to give greater emphasis on equitable provision of health care.

The studies reported here show the diverse ways in which specialists adapted their working patterns to accommodate outreach clinics – some of them replaced NHS clinics, some were carried out in addition and some were private arrangements between the consultants and GPs. None of the studies attempted to measure the disadvantages to hospitals of specialists' absence from the hospital site, though clearly these could be considerable if outreach clinics were to continue to grow.

Different parties stand to gain different things from outreach clinics. These studies focus on benefits for patients – a key element of accountability. However, Gillam's study highlights some of the potential conflicts that arise when outreach clinics are considered in a broader context. This scheme was established for enthusiastic GPs by an entrepreneurial acute trust wanting to increase its market share but the ophthalmologists remained divided about the value of the scheme, and the health authority was constrained by both practical and political considerations from taking a dispassionate stance on the future of the clinics.

CONCLUSION

This book brings together the work of most of the research teams who have been working on specialist outreach clinics during the early and mid-1990s. There is no clear answer to the question 'Are outreach clinics a good idea?' There have been benefits to patients and some costs to the system. Outreach clinics have been popular with GPs but there is continuing concern by specialists that outreach clinics may not represent a cost-effective use of their time and they do not appear to have met their potential in terms of educating either specialists or general practitioners. Even the economic messages from current research are unclear, though it seems unlikely that outreach clinics working to the present model, i.e. fully consultant-led, would be cost-effective if introduced on a very wide scale. However, there may be opportunities to improve services to patients by using outreach clinics, especially if specialist services are viewed as a whole rather than being established on an ad hoc and uncoordinated basis. Outreach clinics may benefit certain groups of patients but they cannot be considered ready for widespread dissemination at present and clinicians and managers should carefully consider the benefits and potential costs of establishing new clinics. A framework for the issues which could be considered, adapted from Leese et al. is shown in Box 7.1.[6]

Box 7.1: Framework of issues to consider when setting-up outreach clinics.

Reasons for setting up outreach clinics
- What is the evidence that a clinic is needed?
- What problems will the outreach clinic solve?
- What specialties have problems?
    - are there lengthy travel times?
    - are there high non-attendance rates?
    - are there problems for particular groups of patients?

Setting up a clinic
- Use current referral patterns to decide on clinic frequency: if they are too infrequent, waiting times may be shorter at hospital clinics; if they are too frequent, will hospital services be adversely affected?
- Can outreach and outpatient clinics be complementary rather than duplicating the same services?
- Will patients from other practices be able to attend the outreach clinic? If so, what additional administrative arrangements will be needed?
- Will patients be consulted about setting up the clinic?

Staff and facilities at the clinic
- Is a room available at an appropriate time?
- Would other clinics have to be cancelled?
- Would practice nurses be involved?
- Would the practice need to buy specific equipment?
- Will extra work be involved for practice staff?

Contracts
- The outreach clinic may not be cheaper. Check details of overheads and future treatment in the contract
- What will happen if clinics are cancelled or there are insufficient referrals?
- Will consultant travel time be included in overall estimate of the 'cost' of the clinic?
- If the outreach clinic is more costly, are there other benefits?
- Will urgent cases referred to the hospital clinic be covered by the same contract?
- What arrangements will there be for tests and other use of hospital facilities?
- How will tests carried out from the practice be paid for?

Box 7.1: Continued.

Implications for GPs
- Will GPs attend the clinic? Will there be other opportunities for learning or increased contact with specialists?
- Will there be guidelines on referral or on numbers of follow-up appointments?
- Will patients be referred to the clinic who would not have been referred to hospital. If so will this be regarded as a benefit or an unnecessary cost?

Implications for trusts and consultants
- Is it appropriate to use outreach clinics defensively against predatory trusts?
- Can outreach clinics be used to gain additional business?
- Will consultant absence affect their teaching or clinical commitments?
- Are limits on outreach clinics needed to prevent unacceptable reduction in hospital services?
- Will the travel time and costs be excessive?
- Will consultants take nursing or junior medical staff to clinics?

REFERENCES

1   Roland M and Wilkin D (1996) Rationale for moving towards a primary care-led NHS. In: *What is the future for a primary care-led NHS?* National Primary Care Research and Development Series, Radcliffe Medical Press Ltd, Oxford.

2   Surender R, Bradlow J, Coulter A, Doll H and Brown SS (1995) Prospective study of trends in referral patterns in fundholding and non-fundholding practices in the Oxford region, 1990–94. *BMJ.* **311**: 1205–8.

3   Audit Commission (1996) *What the doctor ordered: a study of GP fundholders in England and Wales.* HMSO, London.

4   Smith J and Sanderson C (1992) What makes outpatient attendance worthwhile for patients? *Quality Assurance in Health Care.* **4**: 125–32.

5   Gosden T, Black M, Mead N and Leese B The efficiency of specialist outreach clinics in general practice: is further evaluation needed? *Journal of Health Services Research and Policy.* In press.

6   Leese B, Mead N, Black M and Gosden T (1996) Dr Livingstone, I presume? *Health Service Journal.* December 5: 24–6.

Index